DISCLAIMER AND TERMS OF USE AGREEMENT:

(Please Read This Before Using This Book)

This information is not presented by a medical practitioner and is for educational and informational purposes only. The content is not intended to be a substitute for professional medical advice, diagnosis, or treatment. Always seek the advice of your physician or other qualified health provider with any questions you may have regarding a medical condition. Never disregard professional medical advice or delay in seeking it because of something you have read.

Since natural and/or dietary supplements are not FDA approved, they must be accompanied by a two-part disclaimer on the product label: that the statement has not been evaluated by FDA and that the product is not intended to "diagnose, treat, cure or prevent any disease.

The author and publisher of this course and the accompanying materials have used their best efforts in preparing this course. The author and publisher make no representation or warranties with respect to the accuracy, applicability, fitness, or completeness of the contents of this course. The information contained in this course is strictly for educational purposes. Therefore, if you wish to apply ideas contained in this course, you are taking full responsibility for your actions.

The author and publisher disclaim any warranties (express or implied), merchantability, or fitness for any particular purpose. The author and publisher shall in no event be held liable to any party for any direct, indirect, punitive, special, incidental or other consequential damages arising directly or indirectly from any use of this material, which is provided "as is", and without warranties.

As always, the advice of a competent legal, tax, accounting, medical or other professional should be sought. The author and publisher do not warrant the performance, effectiveness or applicability of any sites listed or linked to in this course.

All links are for information purposes only and are not warranted for content, accuracy or any other implied or explicit purpose.

Read all my books on Kindle for free without downloading and printing except you want to buy them.

Contents

A Survival Guide To Overcome And Recover From A Food Allergy

Everyone of us love to eat a variety of food items ranging from fried, grilled, toasted, deep fried, etc. Is your mouth watering when I talk about food items? Hmmm   however, for some people, certain food items would create allergy and they should avoid eating such food items. What is food allergy? It is the immunologic effect that is caused by the existence of food proteins.

A simple search in any of the famous search engines will give you a list of books and materials that details about food allergy. I recently came across a book titled "5 Years without Food: The Food Allergy Survival Guide: How to Overcome Your Food Allergies and Recover Good Healthy." An interesting book that explains what is food allergy and food items that would cause allergy. If you are allergic towards a certain food item, it doesn't mean you will have to forfeit the nutrients that you would have got, am I rite? You also get to understand the food items that can be taken as a supplement or as an alternative. It also explains few treatments related to food allergy. Don't forget to read the book.

Apart from the tips given in the book, I too have listed a few, which would benefit readers who are prone to food allergy.

In general, food items such as shellfish, fish, soya, eggs, peanuts, tree nuts may create allergy in adults. Does it mean kids are not allergic towards food items? Definitely not   Milk, eggs, peanuts are known to create allergies in children. It is always a good idea to be knowledgeable about the food items that are allergic to you.

A key to food items and allergies:

Allergic towards egg: A person who is allergic towards egg is said to be hypersensitive towards nutritional substances derived from eggs such as yolk or the white of egg, albumin, Globulin, eggnog, etc. This may result in overreaction of the immune system.

It is advisable to stay away from food items made with egg if you are allergic towards egg. However, you need not worry about not eating egg. Many substitutes for egg are available in the market today, which includes potato starch, tapioca, etc., and you may use them without any trouble. You can even use apple sauce as an alternative to egg.

Allergic towards tree nuts: What is tree nut allergy? Hypersensitive towards tree nuts is said to be called as tree nut allergy. Don't confuse yourself with tree nuts and peanuts allergy. Both are different. Dry fruits are believed to be tree nuts where as peanuts are legumes. Children are prone to nut allergies than adults.

You can use soy nuts as an alternative to tree nuts. If you are of the opinion that soy nut is a nut, I would like to clarify a point here. It is not a nut, but actually soybean that goes through the procedure of soaking, which is then baked to get the crispy soy nut.

Allergy towards milk substances: Are you allergic towards proteins that are present in cow's milk? If yes, you are allergic towards milk substances.

You may use rice milk or soy milk as a substitute to cow's milk. This way you get the nutrients that you would have got from taking cow's milk.

Allergic towards seafood: Allergy created by the intake of food items such as scaly fishes, crustaceans or shellfishes is termed as allergic towards seafood.

The best way is to stay away from sea foods. If you use a lot of canned food items, ensure that they don't contain ingredients that are made of seafood.

Be picky about the food items that you eat. This may help you surmount the allergic reaction. Certain allergies can be cured in a short period of time; however, you can't treat certain food allergies in your entire life span.

<u>Understanding Common Allergies And Their Symptoms</u>

If you have these sudden attacks of itchiness, asthma, sneezing, coughing, rashes and red spots all over your body, chances are, you are allergic to something. Common allergies and their symptoms can manifest anytime and anywhere so if you have allergic reactions to some types of foods, smell, pollen and others, you need to be very careful and avoid your allergy triggers. Note that some common allergies and their symptoms can cause some complications in your body. Once medical complications happen, danger comes in. To help you understand common allergies and their symptoms, read on.

Types Of Allergies And Their Triggers

Common allergies and their symptoms can be broadly categorized into outdoor and indoor allergy triggers. Both outdoor and indoor allergies can make your life really miserable so be aware of the things that could trigger your allergic reactions. For instance, the most common allergies and their symptoms may be caused by different kinds of pollen. Pollen may come from trees, weeds, grasses and shrubs.

Technically, pollen is a harmless powdery substance that is emitted by the male plants into the air to pollinate the female plants. In other words, pollen is necessary to make plants grow and bear fruits. Unfortunately, there are people who are allergic to this stuff. Since is made up of very tiny particles and can be inhaled by a person, a person who is allergic to this stuff may suffer from different forms of allergies and symptoms.

In most cases, people who are allergic to pollen will suffer from asthma, allergic rhinitis and others. The weather also contributes much to the degree of the sufferings of those people who are allergic to pollen. According to experts, humidity will amplify the allergic reactions of the person. Since the pollen could become trapped in the moisture, it will stay longer in the air and cause more sufferings to people who are allergic to it. During humid conditions the impact of common allergies and their symptoms could magnify, causing the sufferer to feel extremely uncomfortable.

How To Win Your War Against Allergies

On the other hand, while the outdoor allergens may be seasonal, indoor allergens can be an all year round bother. People who are living in windowless apartments and those who are living in polluted areas are especially prone to common allergies and symptoms. Molds and mites are usually the culprit. Since the air in the windowless apartment is recycled, allergens are trapped inside the apartment thus the sufferer may experience an all year round coughing and sneezing.

Food Allergies Can Greatly Diminish Appetite

As much as most people like to eat, it can be depressing to learn they have developed food allergies. Despite how good a particular food may taste it is not worth the potential swelling, itching and the potential for death to consume a food product knowing it can ignite a reaction. While different people may suffer food allergies from different foods, some of the most common are peanuts and shell fish. Most will learn of an allergy the first time they are exposed to it, but allergies develop later in life and may come as a surprise.

When a person consumes a particular food and has an allergic reaction, their best plan is to eliminate that item from their diet. The symptoms of food allergies are very similar other type of allergies and may include runny nose, watering eye as well as a skin rash and hives. Other reactions can include a headache due to sinus infections and pain in the ears as well as diminished hearing.

In some individuals, food allergies can also cause an anaphylactic reaction, which causes a sudden lowering of blood pressure as well as difficulty breathing and in severe cases can lead to death.

Finding The Cause Before It Kills

In most cases, the cause of food allergies can be easy to determine by maintaining a food diary and recording any adverse reactions related to specific foods. Once the list has been narrowed down, any food that causes an allergic reaction should not be eaten. To extract the exact cause of food allergies, the doctor may recommend and skin prick test to determine the cause of allergies before they cause serious health problems.

Many foods contain a multitude of ingredients and it could simply be one of the ingredient causing food allergies and if the product can be found without that ingredient, it will not continue to be a problem. Reading labels in the store can help identify any such ingredients, but can be a problem if eating out in restaurants and establishing the identity of all ingredients may not be possible.

How To Win Your War Against Allergies

The circumstances may be more difficult for children who do not always remember they have food allergies for certain edibles. If they ingest a food that causes a reaction, depending on the level of reaction, they will need to get help quickly to prevent permanent problems. In cases where a child has severe food allergies a medical alert bracelet may be needed to reduce the accidental ingestion of a problem food.

Food Allergy Overview And How To Fight It

Isn't it annoying when you smell the delicious aroma of a meal only to find out that it has an ingredient to which you are allergic? Ah! The demise of every person with food allergies! It is no fun to watch other people devour food that seems so delicious but you can't take part of the experience. How many times have you encountered comments like, great food isn't? And sometimes you just can't bear to admit you are allergic and just smile as if you knew how it tasted.

Then you try to ask questions, what is food allergy? What are causing these annoying symptoms? What's happens inside the body during allergic reactions? Ah! Understanding ones own health condition will better help them accept and overcome whatever's bothering them.

To start with, food allergy is unusual reaction to certain type of food allergen. An allergen is the substance or thing that causes the allergic reactions. Exposure to the allergen sets off the alarm in the human immune system which consequently releases antibodies to fight off the invasion of the perceived foreign body that is the food allergen. It then causes the symptoms you would see when you are in a state of allergic reaction.

The aforementioned is just an overview of the whole picture. Looking more closely, allergic reactions undergo two courses of action. The initial course is the release of immunoglobulin E or IgE by the immune system into the blood stream. IgE is a food-specific antibody and a protein that is the body's immune defense against the food allergen.

Following the initial response is the attachment of the IgE to the mast cells. These mast cells are present in body tissues specially locations of the body where allergic reactions are common. These locations may include the lungs, skin, nasal and oral cavities, and the gastrointestinal system.

As for the food itself, you may have noticed that you are not just allergic to one type of food. There are instances that you experience an allergic reaction to oyster and then later you found out that you are also allergic to crabs and other sea foods. This occurrence is what medical

How To Win Your War Against Allergies

professionals call cross-reactivity, wherein an individual can be allergic to closely related or similar types of foods.

The only way to deal with this unfortunate mishap is to try as best as you can to avoid the foods that set off allergic reactions in your body. There is no cure to food allergy but there are medications out there that can alleviate its symptoms. With the help of a medical health professional, you can be assisted in the ways you can avoid exposures to food allergens. Nutritionists may teach you alternative ingredients or foods to replace the food that will be eliminated from your diet. Also, make it a habit to check food labels for possible ingredients that you may be allergic with and do not hesitate to warn the restaurant employees, like the waiter, about your food allergy to prevent any unwanted accidents.

Individuals who are highly allergic are advised to put on medical alert necklaces or bracelets which declare your condition. As for the medications, some patients who are very vulnerable are also advised to bring with them at all times a self-injectible epinephrine, which is prescribed by the doctor, that can be of great help during sudden attacks of allergic reactions before seeking out for the assistance of an emergency team.

Other medications are antihistamines, bronchodilators, and corticosteroids. Antihistamines help improve symptoms of rhinitis, hives, rashes, and gastrointestinal problems. Corticosteroids alleviate the severity of inflammations of the skin and in other areas of the body. While bronchodilators are utilized to open up air passages of the respiratory tract that has become inflamed which would have resulted to breathing difficulties.

To understand more about your food allergies, you can consult your physician. There are also comprehensive books in the market that can be easily understood by just about anybody that has complete information about food allergies and how to fight it.

<u>Understanding And Preventing Mold Allergies</u>

Allergies are a common ailment among many folks today, and the substances that people are allergic to can vary greatly. For those who are suffering from mold allergies, it may be difficult to cope with the symptoms. The reason that mold allergies can be such a challenge is that there is not a set season for mold to appear, and some sufferers can experience symptoms year-round. The good news is that these types of allergies are relatively rare; when you consider the number of molds that we might be exposed to every day. It is also possible to effectively treat mold allergy symptoms, so you that you do not have to suffer unnecessarily with the sniffling and sneezing that can arise with exposure to the dreaded substance.

Symptoms

The symptoms of mold allergies are similar to those of other allergic reactions, and can include nasal congestion, runny nose, watery eyes, and a skin rash. If you experience these symptoms while raking leaves or mowing grass, you might be suffering from mold allergies. Likewise, if you notice these symptoms when you enter a musty basement or other moist area, mold may indeed be the culprit. To determine if your allergies really are caused by mold spores, you can have an allergy test done at your doctor's office. There are two types of tests that are done; a skin test or a blood sample. Either test can give your doctor a good idea about the substances that you might be allergic to so that he can treat your allergies in the most effective way.

Treatment and Prevention

Treatment for any type of allergy generally includes over the counter medications like decongestants and antihistamines. For more severe symptoms, your doctor can prescribe similar medications in stronger doses. You can also opt for steroidal nasal sprays to keep nasal passages clear, or inhaled medications if you also suffer from asthma. Many of these medications are safe to take over a longer period of time, making them a good option for mold allergy sufferers who might experience symptoms year round.

While there are numerous treatments for allergies that can be very helpful, another good way of reducing symptoms is by prevention. This usually entails an avoidance of the allergy triggers –

How To Win Your War Against Allergies

which in this case would be mold spores. Prevention of mold allergies might include avoiding food that has a greater chance of harboring mold, like cheese and mushrooms, or staying away from damp areas like basements. It is also a good idea to change your furnace filter frequently to prevent mold from developing. With a combination of prevention and treatment options, you can successfully keep your mold allergy symptoms at bay.

Tying Together Allergies And Frequent Urination

People know the common effects of allergies: runny nose, sneezing, itchy eyes or hives. However, there can be a number of different ways your body reacts to an allergic reaction that range from headaches to gastric problems. Having allergies and frequent urination is a symptom many people have not realized exists. It mostly depends on your allergic trigger and your body's sensitivity to it.

Here are a number of a couple of reasons why allergies and frequent urination could occur:

1. Medications - Allergies and frequent urination could be tied to the medicines you are taking. There are many medicines, not just allergy medications that have side effects, one being frequent urination. You could be having an allergic reaction to the medication. Before you stop taking the medication, visit your doctor and rule out any other causes such as a urinary tract infection. If your medicine is a problem, the only way to fix the problem would be to find another prescription that does not cause the same problem but does the same job as the previous medicine.

2. Wheat allergies - Wheat allergies are one of the rarest forms of food allergies, but do exist. When a person is allergic to wheat, they are allergic to the protein in wheat called gluten. A person's body overreacts to the gluten producing a large number of antibodies causing an array of symptoms such cramps, diarrhea and asthma. Wheat allergies and frequent urination have been linked. The only way to help this allergy is by eliminating wheat from your diet. With society becoming more health conscious and offering wheat alternatives, this could be a problem, but your body will thank you for it.

One of the ways to track to see if allergies and frequent urination are related is to keep a food journal. Keep a log of everything you eat and drink in a day. You may find that after you have a particular type of food you are visiting the bathroom more often. This could happen especially with foods and beverages that are acidic such as sodas, coffee and salsa. A detailed journal is important to take with you when visiting your doctor and seeing if allergies and frequent urination are related.

How To Win Your War Against Allergies

Allergies and frequent urination could be a problem if it is affecting your work or personal life. If you notice you are urinating more frequently, visit your doctor.

However, the tie between allergies and frequent urination is not concrete. There are also people who have abnormal reactions to different products, which can cause frequent urination. There is no real rhyme or reason as to why except your body is having an adverse chemical reaction. If you are suffering from frequent urination consult a doctor because there could be a more serious problem such an enlarged prostate, as prostate cancer or a urinary tract infection.

<u>With Allergies Skin Rash Degree Can Vary</u>

Allergic reactions can come in many forms. There is the sneezing with the itchy, watery eyes. Someone can have trouble breathing where their asthma is triggered by a substance in the air. There are many different ways someone can suffer from an allergy. Skin rashes are not rare when it comes to allergic reactions. They can come from all sorts of triggers from food to clothing to laundry detergent. Even going for a stroll in the park, you can walk into something that will give you an allergic skin rash. The key is knowing the difference and taking care of the problem as soon as it happens.

There are different types of skin rashes that can occur from allergies.

Atopic dermatitis: Another name for this is eczema. This allergic skin rash has certain characteristics such as dry, itchy skin. It can be aggravated by clothing, laundry detergent, soaps or stress. Many times it is found in families that have a history of asthma or hay fever. The first way to treat eczema is through proper skin care. Avoid soaps with scents or creams in them. Avoid certain clothing such as wool that can aggravate it. Use warm water when bathing and avoid body lotions with extra ingredients.

Contact dermatitis: This is a skin rash that is caused by coming in contact with a substance that causes a rash on the skin. Another way to get contact dermatitis is by doing that something irritates the skin. Contact dermatitis most commonly happens when a person comes in contact with poison ivy, poison oak or fake jewelry, to name a few, but these are not the only things that can cause it. Contact dermatitis only affects the parts of the skin that were touched. Treatments usually come in the form of topical creams or lotions.

Allergic drug rash: Allergic skin rashes can be caused by having a reaction to medicine. People might have an allergic reaction to drugs and a skin rash will break out. Unfortunately, there is no specific way to test that the skin rash is from an allergy to the medicine. The doctor might recommend the patient stop taking the drugs to see the rash's course of action.

Hives: Anyone who has had hives knows this is terrible allergy. It's a skin rash that can happen on any part of the body. Hives can be caused through other means though and not just an

How To Win Your War Against Allergies

allergy. It can be induced by stress or outside factors. There is no medicine or cream for hives. The itchy, red bumps need to just their course.

Not all skin rashes are allergies. Skin rashes can be caused by other medical conditions. Never self diagnose. Always go to a doctor or a dermatologist to learn the nature of the skin rash. If it does turn out to be an allergic skin rash, visit an allergist and run tests to find out what you are allergic to. This way you can avoid these substances and stop scratching so much.

The Most Common Food Allergies And How To Treat Them

Common food allergies are one of the most popular types of allergies that exist. When you initially eat a food, you may not know you are allergic to it. Minor symptoms of common food allergies usually result in swelling and tingling of the lips and tongue and swelling in the mouth. More severe allergies include trouble breathing, swelling of the throat, vomiting and fainting. These conditions require immediate attention because it could be become fatal. The more common term for these conditions is anaphylaxis shock. People with common food allergies could also suffer from upset stomachs, skin rashes or itchy, swollen eyes. There is no exact symptom that a person with a common food allergy will get so it is important to note all the different reactions you might have after eating a certain meal.

The good thing about common food allergies is that if you stay away from these foods, the allergies will not be a problem. There have been eight foods that are associated with common food allergies.

- Milk
- Eggs
- Peanuts
- Tree nuts
- Fish
- Shellfish
- Soy
- Wheat

About 90 percent of common food allergies can be related to these eight foods. People with these food allergies have gotten help from the Federal Food and Drug Administration identifying harmful foods. Companies and restaurants are required by law to state if any of these foods are in an item. Also, they have to state if one of these foods is used in the cooking process. The FDA is looking out for everyone to make common food allergies uncommon.

How To Win Your War Against Allergies

Reading labels and all warnings on food is important. If you have a peanut allergy, but do not realize that a certain snack could have peanuts in the process, you could end up suffering for a severe reaction. Labels will state if peanuts are or could be used while making the food.

If you think you have a food allergy or notice that after you eat a certain item that you do not feel well, you may want to check with your doctor to see if you have any allergies. There are ways your doctor or an allergist can check for common food allergies. Such tests include a blood test, skin test and a careful description of what you have eaten. It is smart to keep a journal of foods and write down whenever you have a reaction. This way doctors can use this when deciphering the information and will be able to tell if you have a common food allergy.

If you do have common food allergies, let your doctor know on every visit about this allergy. There are some medications that you might not be able to take because you might have a reaction to the medicine.

What Your Doctors Know About Dairy Allergies

Dairy allergies are not fun to deal with. Those with this allergy can testify to the pain and general inconvenience dairy allergies cause. Symptoms to dairy allergies range from moderate to severe with some of the more common symptoms being diarrhea, vomiting and a skin rash. People with asthma might begin wheezing after having a dairy product, which is classified as products containing milk.

What are Dairy Allergies?

Dairy allergies occur when your body has an adverse reaction to a protein found in these products. It is actually one of the most common food allergies. Babies who suffer from dairy allergies many times out grow the allergy once they reach three years of age. However, parents still need to be careful and keep a constant vigil over their children and their reaction to foods.

Treatment of Dairy Allergies

Unfortunately, for dairy allergy sufferers the only way to avoid dairy allergies is by avoiding the products. There are no special pills to make the body less reactive. People should avoid milk, butter, cheese and all types of cream. Read the nutritional label and check for anything that could be harmful. There are other ingredients that states a product uses dairy milk: whey, casein, lactic acid and sodium lactate. If one does ingest a dairy product, there are ways to combat the allergic reaction. Sometimes an Epinephrine pen is used if the allergy is severe and needs immediate attention. Otherwise an antihistamine, more commonly known as Benedryl, could be prescribed to subside the allergic reaction.

Alternatives to Milk

There are many replacements made readily available for people suffering from dairy allergies. You can find rice milk, soy milk, almond milk and other variations in the supermarket. However, these types of milk are not suitable for a child's nutrition. Get a doctor's recommendation on where to get calcium and other nutrients you are missing out on from dairy products. Children need extra attention to get the proper nutrition. Look for juice drinks with added calcium and other products that could help.

Difference Between Allergies and Lactose Intolerance

Dairy allergies shouldn't be confused with being lactose intolerant. These are two different problems. If someone suffers from dairy allergies, the body is having an adverse chemical reaction to the protein found in milk products. In a lactose intolerant person, the body cannot process the sugar found in milk because of the absence of lactase in a person's body. This is a non-allergy reaction. People who are lactose intolerant will also have different symptoms that are mostly intestinal related: flatulence, stomach cramps, bloating and diarrhea.

Consider Fluconazole For Mold Allergies

Allergies that never go away might be a sign of a bigger problem or caused by a substance that has not been explored yet. If the sneezing does not stop and the runny nose continues, perhaps it is not the pollen in the air. You may want to look into mold. Mold can be a dangerous substance, not just an annoyance. To help with the allergies, a doctor might prescribe fluconazole for mold allergies. Fluconazole is also known as Diflucan.

What is a Mold Allergy?

Let's start with defining a mold allergy. Mold allergies occur when microscopic fungal spores cause allergies when inhaled. The spores are so tiny that they get past the nasal defenses and get into the lungs. Mold can be found anywhere in the home. However, the places where mold is more common are in damp basements, closets and bathrooms. Anywhere where there is moisture, there is a possibility for mold. It does not have to be just inside the home. Mold can grow in the garden or yard. So if you are having constant allergy problems you may want to check to see if there is mold. Talk to a doctor about the possibility of getting fluconazole for mold allergies.

Symptoms of Mold Allergies

Mold allergy symptoms might be difficult to figure out because they are so like many other common allergies. You have to deal with sneezing, runny nose, coughing and postnasal drip. There is not a simple way to tell if you have a mold allergy. A doctor will need to swab your nose and send it out to a lab to be tested for mold. Lab tests will be able to tell what type of mold is causing your allergies.

Treatment of mold allergies

There are a few ways to deal with mold allergies. When you find out that your allergies are due to mold, the first step you want to take is removing the mold from your home. It is the only way mold allergies are going to ever end. In the meantime, discuss with your doctor medications such as fluconazole for mold allergies. Fluconazole for mold allergies comes in pill and liquid

How To Win Your War Against Allergies

form to make ingestion easier for the patient. Fluconazole deals with many different problems in the fungi family, which is why it is so durable for mold allergies.

There might be side effects to the drug, so check with your doctor. Side effects of fluconazole for mold allergies could include nausea, diarrhea and loss of appetite. Those taking medications for diabetes, insomnia or high blood pressure might want to avoid fluconazole for mold allergies. There could be adverse reactions to other medications you are taking.

Common Peanut Allergies Can Cause Fatal Reaction

What Are Peanut Allergies?

Peanut allergies occur when a person's body has an adverse reaction peanuts or peanut-containing products. A person's immune system tries to fight off the peanut as it does not recognize it as a substance that is not harmful. The scary thing about peanut allergies is that it is the most common cause of life-threatening allergic reactions in the United States. This is a very serious and dangerous allergy and should be treated carefully. Those who suffer from peanut allergies need to vigilante with the types of foods that they eat.

Symptoms of Peanut Allergies

Symptoms range from moderate to severe, but either way should be treated immediately. A person can suffer from itching, swelling, nausea or abdominal cramps. However, it can get worse than that, much worse. Many who have peanut allergies have shortness of breath, wheezing and can loss consciousness (anaphylaxis). You can also develop hives over your body. Usually, symptoms occur within just a few minutes of exposure to peanuts, but there have been cases where it took hours. If a person does suffer from the most serious of symptoms, anaphylaxis, they require immediate attention. They will have difficulty breathing, their blood pressure will drop and could have seizures.

Foods to Avoid

The problem is in the food that we eat. There are many foods out there that are made with peanuts or cooked in peanut oil. Labels now have to state if a product contains or can contain nuts even if there are not any nuts readily seen in the food. Peanut allergies are so severe, the FDA requires food and restaurant companies to state if a food has nuts in them. Obvious foods to avoid are peanut butter, granola bars, cookies, other types of nuts and energy bars. But take a closer look at some of the other foods a person who has peanut allergies might come in contact with. There are some sauces and salad dressings that are made from crushed nuts. Many baked goods have nuts in them including cookies, cakes, marzipan. Check potato chips or salty food packages to see if the food was made in peanut oil.

How To Win Your War Against Allergies

Treatment of Peanut Allergies

Depending on the severity of the symptoms, a person can have either an antihistamine (Benadryl) or an emergency injection of epinephrine. Those who know they suffer an extreme case of peanut allergies should carry epinephrine with them at all times. But the only way to not suffer from peanut allergies is to avoid peanuts and all the potential harmful foods as well. If a person thinks they suffer from a peanut allergy, they should see a doctor or allergist who can perform a battery of tests to tell what specific substances a person is allergic to including if they have peanut allergies.

How To Cope With Seasonal Allergies

Anyone who suffers from seasonal allergies knows how daunting spring can be. The flowers are in bloom, the birds are coming back from their southern vacation and you can't stop sneezing. There is nothing like a cool, spring morning when the pollen count is so high, you can't go outside or you will suffer from sneezing, itchy, watery eyes and an itchy throat. Seasonal allergies -- your worse nightmare.

The routine is the same every year and the medicine cabinet is filled with anti-allergy medication. There are those who suffer differently from season allergies. While the common symptoms affect many people, seasonal allergies are worse in people who suffer from asthma and allergic rhinitis. Seasonal allergies aren't just an inconvenience anymore, but become a medical problem. People are hospitalized every year from seasonal allergies.

There are ways to help yourself to make the seasonal changes easier.

- Eating essential fatty acids is one of the ways to lower the symptoms from seasonal allergies. Studies that have been done have showed that essential fatty acids and flaxseed help reduce allergic reactions in many people. Increase your daily dose of these essential fatty acids.

- Get extra Vitamin C. This vitamin can lower the amount of histamine found in the blood. Eat lots of fruits and vegetables that contain vitamin C to ward off any potential problems. You can even help your body fight off any colds.

- Monitor pollen and mold counts. If you keep a close eye on the pollen and mold counts, you will know when it is safe to venture outdoors. Keep the windows and doors sealed tight to prevent seasonal allergies. However, check the house for mold as well. These can keep your allergies going if there is mold in the house.

- Wash clothes when coming in from the outside during pollen season. The pollen that sets off your seasonal allergies is the microscopic kind. You can't see it, but it gets into your system, which is what drives your body crazy. If you were gardening or went for a walk, take off

How To Win Your War Against Allergies

the clothes you were wearing and wash them as soon as possible. This will help with keeping the pollen at bay.

- Wash your hair before bed. If you were outside during the day, pollen could be trapped in your hair. What you don't want is the pollen going from your hair to your pillow. At that point, you are doomed because you will suffer from seasonal allergies all night long. Wash your hair before going to bed to ensure a good night's sleep.

Seasonal allergy sufferers don't have to be discouraged any time a brand new season starts. There are ways to prevent seasonal allergies and tricks to make the allergy season more bearable.

Skin Allergies Account For Most Complaints

Skin Allergies are different for every person. Someone who gets a skin allergy can get it in a confined area or over their entire body. There are even times when a person can get them on their hands and feet, making it difficult to do every day tasks. When a person gets a skin allergy, it's called allergic contact dermatitis. The skin has a chemical reaction to the substance it has come into contact with. In these cases, you have to physically touch it to get the allergy. Some of the culprits may even surprise you.

Testing for Skin Allergies

One way to figure out what causes skin allergies is by playing a guessing game. However, there are no winners in this one. You would test products on your skin to see if have a reaction. Don't worry, there is an easier way. Doctors will do patch testing. They take a small piece of skin (this doesn't hurt) and then put each patch of skin in contact with the common allergens. They look to see if there is a reaction. The doctors do all the hard work for you and you don't have to suffer.

These are some of the most common causes of skin allergies:

- ***Nickel and gold.*** These metals are usually found in jewelry. The nickel is found in clasps or buttons. Gold is a little more common. Many pieces are made or plated with gold. If you have an allergy to either of these metals, usually a rash will break out where the metal touched your skin. Many people tend to have a reaction to costume jewelry.

- ***Balsam of Peru.*** This fragrance is found in many lotions and perfumes. Another name for it is myroxylon pereirae. If this is the culprit of your skin allergy, check the ingredients in perfumes and lotions you use to see if this is present.

- ***Neomycin sulfate.*** This substance is commonly found in first aid creams and ointments. Unfortunately, a doctor might prescribe a topical cream for a previous skin rash, only for the patient to find out they also have skin allergies to this substance. It can also be found in cosmetics, soap and pet food.

How To Win Your War Against Allergies

- Bacitracin. This is a topical antibiotic. Some people might use it on cuts or burns.

- Cobalt chloride. This is a real problem for some people because this is normally found in antiperspirants. However, there are other places cobalt chloride shows up such as hair dye and pieces plated in it (buttons, snaps, tools).

- Quaternium 15. This is a preservative found in many products than women tend to use. It can be found in self tanners, shampoo, nail polish and sunscreen. Try to find products that do not use this if you have skin allergies to Quaternium 15.

What You Should Know About Sun Allergies

Sun allergies can be a dangerous reaction to the sun especially when many people who suffer from sun allergies don't even know they have it. Sun allergies can resemble sunburn. This is why many people don't even realize that they are allergic to sunlight. This is commonly called photosensitivity.

There are some things to look for, though. If you are outside for only a few minutes and already notice redness to exposed parts of your body, you want to be careful when outdoors. Try to cover up these parts of the body by wearing loose, light fitting clothing, a hat and staying in the shade. Some of the more common places are the hands, forearms, legs and back of the neck. The rashes could be itchy or burning and last for a few days. It can go away by itself, or you may need to see a doctor. Treatments for sun allergies range from oral beta-carotene to topical creams. Some more severe cases can include blisters or hives over the body. You should be especially careful if you develop these symptoms on parts of the body that were clothed, like your chest and back.

A doctor may perform some more serious tests such as a biopsy or blood test to rule out any other problems. There are also medications and lotions that can make the skin more susceptible to sun allergies. Read the label of all products to be safe.

There is a difference between sunburn and sun allergies. Sunburns occur when the body's protective skin pigment can't protect the skin well enough from ultraviolet light. When you have an allergy to sunlight, your body's immune system reacts against it. This is what causes the breakout on your skin.

To avoid sun allergies, just a follow a few simple tips:

1. Don't go outside during peak sunlight hours (10 a.m. to 4 p.m.). Your body will have a quicker reaction at this time of day.
2. Don't deliberately sunbathe, even in tanning beds. Those with sun allergies won't be happy with the results.
3. Apply sunscreen 20 minutes before going outdoors. Apply it every two hours, after swimming and working out.

How To Win Your War Against Allergies

4. Dress properly. Wear light clothing, wide-brimmed hats and sunglasses.

Remember, even if you do not suffer from sun allergies, you should always be safe while outdoors. You can get skin cancer and wrinkles from over exposure to the sun. Wear sunscreen and don't stay outside during peak sunlight hours longer than you have to.

Tattoo Allergies – An Uncommon But Real Problem

Tattoos are becoming a popular trend these days. Anyone can have a tattoo, even the most unlikely of people. However, with the onset of the tattoo craze, a problem has emerged -- tattoo allergies.

The ink in the artwork contains ingredients that cause the tattoo allergies. The most common allergen is found in red and yellow ink. The problem with tattoo ink is that it is unregulated. Almost anything can be used to create the pigments that make up the ink. Some of the more common ingredients include nickel, mercury (although less and less), cobalt and cadmium.

Signs of the allergy include itchiness around and on the tattoo, raised bumps, redness, irritation or hives. Worse case scenarios include pussing and oozing around the tattoo and sores. When this occurs, the person has to see a doctor immediately. Usually, a steroid will be given at the site of the problem that will eliminate the allergy.

Just because you get a tattoo and do not have a reaction a week later does not mean you are in the clear. Tattoo allergies sometimes do not show up right away. There have been cases where the allergy did not show up until years later. Usually, there is something that triggered the reaction to take place such as another tattoo (creating more exposure), change in weather or even a sickness. The treatment at this point is the same.

If the allergy is severe, the ink can be removed by a doctor using a laser. If the allergy is not that bad where you just suffer from occasional itching or swelling, over the counter anti-inflammatory and anti-histamine creams should do the trick. If you ever noticed that during the summer months, your tattoo gets itchy or a little red, this could be due to a tattoo allergy. Most people who do have this moderate reaction tend to just deal with the problem.

Unfortunately, there is no way of knowing you are going to have tattoo allergies. There are no tests that can be done beforehand. You can't have a small piece of skin that is out of the way tested because of the length of time some tattoo allergies take to appear. The only time people find out they have a tattoo allergy is after the tattoo is already on their body.

How To Win Your War Against Allergies

Take careful consideration on what the tattoo artist tells you about cleaning your tattoo. This prevents any immediate reactions your body may have and also an easier way to watch for signs of an allergic reaction. Keep in mind tattoo allergies are rare, so don't shy away from them if you really want to get one.

<u>Reactions To Allergies May Be Nothing To Sneeze At</u>

Most doctors and researchers are still quite confused as to why certain things cause allergies in some people. Many a times some people react to certain things triggering off a series of reactions in their bodies while the same things may not have any effect on others .It is often difficult to pinpoint the exact reason why someone is having an allergy to a particular thing while the same thing may have no reaction on another person. With allergies it is difficult to find out what exactly is causing them and dealing with these symptoms can be really tough. An allergy can be anything from a sneeze to a running nose, or even an anaphylactic shock which can even lead to death.

Doctors are of the opinion that when immunity is down in a person it means that they are prone to allergies. The immune system in a person when it perceives that an alien object is harmful to the body, it gets ready to fight off the intruder and so begins to produce a number of symptoms like hives or rashes on the skin, running nose, watering eyes and sneezing .The moment the alien object leaves the body the symptoms of allergy which the person had also subsides but there are also times when they can take more time to subside.

Many a time allergies are a disadvantage to many people. For example, people who are allergic to hair will find that they cannot have a pet dog or cat as the hair from the animal's body can trigger off a series of chain reactions in their body.

There are ways to prevent certain allergies. Many people are allergic to dust and so any sweeping or dusting would immediately cause reactions in their body. Pollens from flowers are also known to cause allergies. By using a vacuum cleaner which has an inbuilt filter it is possible for us to remove dust and dust mites from our surrounding areas and we can also fit filtering systems to protect us from air borne pollens coming from outside.

Though there are many tests to determine the causes of allergies, the skin prick test is by far the best. This test is best conducted under the supervision of an allergy specialist. Here what the doctor does is inject each and every item they feel is causing allergy into the patient's body. This helps the doctors to narrow down on what exactly is causing the allergy.

How To Win Your War Against Allergies

There are many allergy medications which patients can take so that they can do their work normally. There are also medications which can stop the allergy even before it causes an attack. It is always better to test for allergies before you decide to take any particular medication for it.

<u>Understanding Common Allergies And Their Symptoms</u>

Many a times we find that we begin to sneeze for no reason, develop sudden rashes all over the body, begin to itch all over, begin to gasp for breath, or start coughing. Don't worry as all these just indicate that we are allergic to something. Many people suffer from common allergies and the symptoms for these can just about show up anywhere anytime. We have to be especially careful if we are allergic to certain types of foods, pollens and smells as these can easily trigger allergies in us. It is advisable that we take ample precautions to avoid these allergies by consciously being aware of them. Common allergies can cause complications in people so it is better if take precautions to avoid them.

There are many items or objects both inside and outside the home which can cause allergies to many people. So it is wiser that we be alert about the possible things that may trigger allergies in us. A very common thing which causes allergies in most people is pollen which can come from flowers, trees, shrubs and plants.

Pollen by itself is quite harmless and it is actually a powdery substance that male plants send out into the atmosphere to pollinate female plants. Pollens play an important part in plants bearing fruits and their growth. Though it is important for the plants, it is not so for humans as it can cause allergies. People when they happen to inhale these tiny particles of powdery substance find that they begin to either gasp for breath or start to sneeze.

Inhalation of pollen mostly causes an asthmatic attack or allergic rhinitis in a person. The weather also further contributes to worsen the allergy. Experts are of the opinion that when the weather is moist it further makes it worse. This is because the pollen gets trapped in the moist air and remains in the atmosphere for a longer period causing more attacks. That is why many people who suffer from allergies find that they become worse during cold weather.

Outdoor allergens are only seasonal while the allergens indoors are there throughout the year. Those people who live cooped up in apartments with no windows and in areas which are highly polluted will find that they are more prone to allergies. This is because of the continuous presence of molds and mites in such places. The congested air which does not get to circulate gets trapped in the same place causing the person living there to have allergic reactions all the time.

Causes And Treatments Of Eye Allergies

When we say allergies we normally refer to only symptoms like itching, running nose, sneezes and hives. We never associate allergies to eyes too. Allergies not only affect the sinus and nasal cavities but they also make the eyes to start itching by making them to swell, turn red and begin to water. Eye allergies can also be treated effectively by simple medications. Prevention is better than cure so it is better that we learn how to protect ourselves from eye allergies first. We must also know why they occur and how to treat them.

Our eyes are important organs which are continuously exposed to the outside all the time that we are awake. Because of continuous exposure the eyes are more susceptible to allergens attacking them and that's why more people get affected easily. Unlike the nose and its passage way where you can find tiny hairs called cilia which help to filter all the harmful bacteria, the eyes do not have such in built protection. Because of this the eyes are more prone to being attacked by harmful bacteria which is always lurking around in the air and causing allergies in the eyes.

If you are someone who is already suffering from allergies of any kind then you can be sure that you will also suffer from eye allergies. So if you have sneezes due to the pollens during the moist season then are sure that you will also have eye allergies. If you also have a family history of allergies or have atrophic dermatitis you are sure to suffer from eye allergies. But do not get disheartened because there are various treatments available that can be used for treating eye allergies.

Now what are the treatments for eye allergies you may wonder? The best way you can avoid eye allergies is through prevention. If you are aware of what to avoid then you can be sure that you will not be susceptible to it. If you feel that your hands have come into contact with a known allergen then make sure that you avoid rubbing or touching your eyes with those hands. Many people tend to rub their eyes with their hands not realizing that it is one of the main causes for allergies. If you still feel that by taking all precautions necessary that you still seem to have itching and watery eyes then it would be advisable to take medications. These medications can be bought over the counter or you can get your doctor to prescribe them for you. These

How To Win Your War Against Allergies

medications are mainly eye drops which have to be applied to the eyes a couple of times in a day.

It is difficult to cope with eye allergies as they are very uncomfortable and irritating to the eyes, so it is best that you talk to our doctor to find ways to reduce allergy symptoms in the eyes.

Food Allergies Can Greatly Diminish Appetite

Everyone loves to eat but most are unaware of the fact the food they have can cause allergies. Foods can look attractive and be tasty too but it certainly is not worth the trouble when we consume such food and discover that we are allergic to them. Food allergies can cause swelling, itching and even death in some cases. Different types of foods can have different reactions in people. Foods like peanuts, and shell fish are known to cause allergies in many people. It is only after they have eaten it for the first time that many people discover that they are allergic to it. People can also develop allergies much later in their lives due to these foods. The best way to avoid an allergic reaction to a particular food is to avoid the food that caused it in the first place. Though most of the symptoms of food allergies are similar to other allergies like running nose, swelling and watering of eyes, rashes and hives, other symptoms could be headaches caused by sinus infections, hearing problems with pain in the ears. Some food allergies can cause people to have anaphylactic attacks and even be the cause of sudden lowering of their blood pressure, breathing problems and even death.

Those who are allergic to certain foods should first determine what foods are causing allergic reactions in their bodies. Once they have made a list of the foods which they think is causing allergies in them they should avoid those foods in their diet. The doctor would be helpful in helping you to determine the exact food that is causing allergic reactions in your body by getting you to take a skin prick test.

Foods are made up of many ingredients and any one of these could be causing the allergies. So it is best to find out which ingredient is actually causing the allergy so that you can avoid it totally. In supermarkets you can read the labels on the food packets and find out if the particular ingredient that is causing food allergy to you is present. If it is present then it is best to avoid that food. But this is not possible when you eat in restaurants.

Children are the biggest sufferers of food allergies as they normally fail to remember what causes allergies in them and consume the food. If such children have an allergic reaction it is best to get help quickly so that it does not worsen further. A child who is prone to food allergies should wear a medical alert bracelet so that they can be saved if they accidentally consume foods that can cause allergies to them.

Treating Fruit Allergies

Fruits are very important in a diet as they supply all the vitamins, minerals and fiber that the body needs to maintain strength and health. But not everyone is able to consume fruit as some people find that taking fruits can cause allergic reactions in their bodies. The allergic reactions which fruits cause can be easily recognized and it is always quite easy to say which fruit is allergic to a person. So once the fruit is identified as causing an allergy the person can best avoid the fruit.

Oral allergy syndrome is very common to fruit allergies as consuming a certain fruit will cause swellings in certain parts like the tongue, mouth, lips and throat etc. The moment the fruit comes into contact with our mouth or lips they begin to burn or swell.

This syndrome is not restricted to fruits alone but also vegetables. Many people display the same allergic symptoms when they eat certain vegetables. This is caused by the chemical reactions which take place between the pollens and proteins. It is common that people who have fruit allergies are also allergic to pollens. Only when the fruits and vegetables are eaten fresh do they cause allergies in people not when they are cooked and eaten. This is because the pollens and proteins which are present get destroyed when cooked.

Some of the other symptoms which fruit allergies cause are skin irritations, redness and rashes or hives. Sometimes due to fruit allergies the blood pressure can also drop drastically cutting off oxygen supply to the brain. The mouth throat and airways begin to swell restricting air to the lungs and this leaves the person gasping for breath which in turn leads to death.

We sometimes notice that only certain classes of fruits tend to cause allergies to us. Like for instance if we are allergic to rag weed then we will find that when we eat fruits like bananas, and melons like watermelon, cantaloupe and honeydew will also cause allergy reactions.

In the case of Birch tree allergy you will find certain fruits like apples, pears, cherries, kiwi and stone fruit which are more likely to cause allergies also. Certain other fruits like lemons, oranges limes and grapefruit which belong to the citrus variety can also cause allergies. This is mainly due to the acidic nature of the citrus fruits which cause allergic reactions.

How To Win Your War Against Allergies

The best way to avoid fruit allergies is not to eat those fruits so that all that rashes, swelling and skin irritations can be avoided. There are people who have become resistant to fruit allergies because of the allergy injections which they have taken. Though there is another option which is to have the fruits cooked and eaten to avoid allergic reactions in your body.

Lake Water Allergies: Understanding Swimmer's Itch

Most people cannot resist themselves when they see a nice clear pond or lake. They immediately get out of their clothes and jump or wade into the water to have a refreshing swim. What they do not realize is that there many be allergens inside the water which can cause serious problems to their skin. Doctors have found that swimming in such contaminated water can cause discomforts and skin allergies which may leave scars too.

This is what is known as lake water allergies or swimmer's itch. The water in lakes and ponds can be contaminated and this will cause allergic reactions leading to infections on the skin. By contamination it is not meant that they may contain harmful chemical substances which have been released from industries but that which is caused by the animals and birds living around the water body. These birds and animals come to the water bodies to drink water and sometimes even for a swim.

Many of the lakes and ponds carry parasites from birds and animals which are released in to the water especially during summer season when these animals come to the water bodies to drink water. We must understand that the ponds and lakes being the natural habitat of these creatures it is not possible to drive them away and it is up to us humans to stay away from such places and refrain from taking a swim if you are someone prone to allergies.

The symptoms which you can develop if you swim in contaminated water are that your skin begins to burn, itch and start tingling just a few hours after your swim. There are some people whose body will react 12 hours after the swim and develop red pimples all over the body soon after the swim. These nasty pimples can develop into serious blisters if they are not treated quickly. These symptoms will cause plenty of discomfort for a week or so before it actually subsides and can be painful too. Make sure to apply anti allergy creams which will help the blisters to subside and you will be saved from having to go to the hospital.

Some people suffer from more serious problems which can occur due to lake allergies. And this is further aggravated if you continuously expose your body to the contaminated water. Serious symptoms like shortness of breath, fever, nasty skin lesions must be treated immediately and this can cause further complications, so seeing a doctor would be the best thing to do.

<u>Understanding And Preventing Mold Allergies</u>

Most people suffer from different types of allergies due to various allergens and one of them is mold allergies. One of the most problematic of allergies is due to molds as this is one allergy that can occur at any time as there is no fixed season for molds to appear. This makes it miserable for those suffering from mold allergies as they will never know when they are likely to get one. But the number of people who suffer from mold allergies is far less than the other allergies though more mold can be found in everyday life. Mold allergies tend to cause sneezing and watery eyes in people and these symptoms can be effectively treated with medication and even prevention.

Mold allergies have the same symptoms as that of other allergies. The common symptoms of mold allergies are nasal congestion, running nose, watery eyes, and rashes or hives on the skin. If you have been in the garden raking the leaves or mowing the grass and you suddenly find that you begin to sneeze continuously and start to itch all over the body then be sure that you are indeed suffering from mold allergies. Sometimes you may even suffer from these symptoms when you enter a musty basement or any place that is moist. To confirm and verify that you are indeed suffering from mold allergies it is best that you see your doctor immediately and have an allergy test done. Normally there are two different types of tests that are carried out. One is the blood test and the other is a skin test. The results of either of the tests will help your doctor determine what exactly is causing your allergy and what medication he or she can give you.

The treatments for most allergies are the prescription of anti histamines and decongestants. If it is more severe then your doctor will prescribe a stronger dosage. To clear your congested nose you can use steroidal sprays or inhalers incase you suffer from asthma. All these medications have been found to be extremely safe and so for mold allergy sufferers, it is not harmful for them to take it all year long.

Though there are medications for such allergies a more effective way is to prevent it. The best way would be to avoid that which can cause the allergy which is the mold spores. Stay away from foods which can develop molds much easily like mushroom and cheese and also stay away from damp places like the basements if you want to avoid mold allergies. Mold can also form on furnace filters, so changing them regularly would prevent molds from forming. Prevention and treatment are ideal ways to tackle mold allergies.

Nasal Allergies

If you are prone to sneezing problems then blame it on your genetics and your body's lack of immunity. Allergic rhinitis or nasal allergy is bound to occur in a person if they are exposed to allergens, pollution, and cigarette smoke or happen to have a low weight at birth.

Doctors are puzzled as to why some people are allergic to certain substances while others are not, but one thing they are sure is that your body responds to these allergens. Your body's immune system has been programmed in such a way as to react whenever a foreign body gets into the nose and these triggers off a series of reactions in the body when the immune system begins its fight to repel the substance. During this process a chemical substance called histamine is released. This is why your eyes begin to water and your nose starts running. At times more severe problems like wheezing and breathing difficulties occur in some people.

Many a times it is allergens which are present in the atmosphere that are the main cause for nasal allergies though these allergens can come from different sources. One of the main causes of nasal allergies through out the country is due to pollens, and their concentration can vary according to the places. Some places may be concentrated with flowering varieties which can generate enough pollen in the air while it may not be so in other places. Some pollen like rag weed can travel far and wide, so even if you live in a city you may still be affected by it. Flowering trees, plants, grass and bushes can also release a number of pollen grains into the air causing nasal allergies.

Though dust can cause you to sneeze it may not cause nasal allergy. But dust mites which are tiny microscopic organisms which can be found in mattresses, carpets and furniture can cause nasal allergy. You will know for sure that it is the dust mites which are actually causing you to sneeze when in the winter months the pollens in the air are at a minimal and you still find yourself sneezing endlessly.

Another serious allergic problem is caused by animal dander. Dander which comes from pets like dogs and cats easily settle down in carpets and furniture and cause you to experience sneezing problems even after you have got rid of your pets. The only way that you can get rid of dander once and for all is getting the carpet and upholstery in the sofas in your home vacuumed thoroughly and having them shampooed.

How To Win Your War Against Allergies

You will know that you are having a nasal allergy the moment your nose starts to twitch and you begin sneezing for no reason. It is the body's way of trying to get rid of the allergen. The nose then starts to run and this is how the body's mechanism tries to wash out the allergen. A little later say after a few hours you will find that you are now having a stuffy nose and you become extremely sensitive to other irritants. You will have to endure this for the duration it takes for the body to have the allergen to be cleared from your body. For some people they can develop more serious problems like asthma or sinus infections.

<u>Symptoms Of Allergies: When To Seek Medical Help</u>

We must know when to seek medical help just incase we suffer from any form of allergy symptoms. We normally never know when we are going to be stricken with an allergy. Common symptoms of allergies are running nose, sneezing, watery eyes, itching and hives on the skin. Allergies can strike anyone anytime and just about anywhere if the allergens are around. So you will never know when you are going to have that sneeze or itching. Most allergies can be treated easily using over the counter medications, homeopathic medications and even by just avoiding the triggers. But there are certain allergies which can be life threatening if not treated immediately. This can even cause death to the person if the symptoms are severe. This is the reason why we should understand the difference between allergies whose symptoms can be classified as mild, moderate and severe and when medical help should be sought.

The symptoms which can be termed mild are those which we normally experience like sneezing, watery eyes, itching and nasal congestion. Sometimes there might even be rashes on the skin or hives. Sometimes the symptoms do not spread all over the body and can be termed as very mild. If you find the rashes spreading all over your body then you are in for a more serious problem. These types of mild symptoms can be treated using nasal decongestants, eye drops, anti histamines and topical creams for the hives or rashes. These would not warrant a visit to a doctor but only when the symptoms last more than 2 weeks.

Allergy symptoms can be termed to be moderate to severe if the symptoms spread all over the body and when they become threatening to the patient's life. Symptoms like continuous itching and difficulty in breathing can be termed as moderate while severe symptoms include swelling in different parts of the body which can even cause discomfort while swallowing food or breathing problems. Sometimes nausea, diarrhea and vomiting can also occur when it is severe. At times one can even feel dizzy with no clarity of thoughts. The moment you find yourself suffering from any of these symptoms then seeking immediate medical help is important and advisable. These are the symptoms or the life threatening condition called anaphylaxis.

Normally most allergies that occur in people are often mild and can be quite easily treated using over the counter prescriptions or home remedies. But having a knowledge about the severity of allergic symptoms will not be harmful either as it will help you to seek immediate medical help if the situation warrants one.

How To Live With Wheat Allergies

It is quite common to find many children suffering from food allergies these days. Various foods can cause different types of allergies and the symptoms can also vary from mild to moderate to severe. It has been found that wheat is one of the top eight foods which cause allergies. Most of the food that is available contains wheat as an ingredient in one form or the other. Normally we find that it is children who are the main sufferers of wheat allergies though they soon outgrow them but sometimes even some adults tend to suffer from wheat allergies too.

The time taken for wheat allergy to show up after the food is eaten is normally anywhere between a few minutes to a few hours and the symptoms also can be anywhere between mild and severe. Anaphylaxis is a life threatening allergy symptom which needs immediate medical help. The common symptoms for wheat allergy include nasal congestion, swelling of the air way and inflammation, irritations on the skin or hives, or even nausea, vomiting and diarrhea. When the symptoms are more severe then the person can experience shock, dizziness, rapid pulse and constriction of the airways. Anyone found suffering from these symptoms would need immediate medical help as it can be life threaten.

If you find that you are suffering from wheat allergies than the best way is to avoid all wheat products in your diet. This will reduce your chances of getting an allergic reaction. The more the reactions the more severe the allergy is and therefore it is advisable to see your doctor immediately even if you find a mild symptom. Your doctor will then carry out a series of tests to find out if wheat was really the culprit for the allergy. Once it is verified that it is wheat which is the cause for the allergy than you will be advised to avoid all wheat products. You too will find it easier to avoid wheat products from your diet as most US manufacturers make it a point to list the ingredients on their food packages.

If you have a severe wheat allergic reaction your doctor would advise you to take what is called the Epipen treatment. In this treatment which is done as an emergency measure for wheat allergies an injection is given. You can also wear am bracelet which alerts people around you about your wheat allergy problems if you do happen to eat some wheat product by mistake. Wheat allergy sufferers are normally told to avoid all wheat products in their diets and to take anti histamine if by chance they get stricken by the allergy. Wheat allergies occur more commonly in children than in adults and even children tend to outgrow their wheat allergies as they grow up.

How To Win Your War Against Allergies

This Product Is Brought To You By

DAVID A OSEI